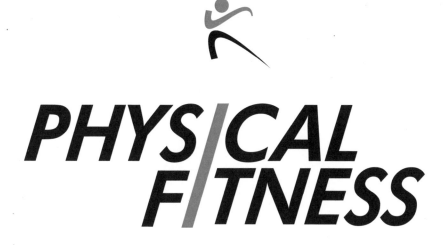

PHYS|CAL F|TNESS

XBX 12-Minute Plan for Women

First published in Great Britain in 2015 by:

BX Plans Ltd
Remus House
Coltsfoot Drive
Peterborough
PE2 9BF
United Kingdom

ISBN 978-1-91084-300-0

Contents

Foreword

We just don't walk enough anymore. Wheels take us everywhere we want to go, whether on a long trip or just half a mile, or even less. Yet we still want to eat plenty, often consuming far more calories than we burn in exercise. There are gyms of course, but they can be expensive, and you have to sign up often months ahead. The gym may not be nearby, so there is the time spent just getting there and back to take into consideration, as well as the extra fuel costs. But you want to be fit and know that taking regular exercise will improve your health; you haven't time for long country walks... So how do you go about getting as fit as possible?

The exercises contained in this book are your answer. They don't require expensive equipment, just your body and enough room to stretch and turn. They were designed originally by the Royal Canadian Air Force, and are meant to ensure that even after a relatively prolonged period of inactivity you can spring quickly into action when required.

They are designed for those with sedentary jobs, perhaps who are city dwellers who aren't particularly interested in joining a sports' club or taking part in organised sport. We all have to run for a bus from time to time, or chase a toddler heading for the gate, so we need to be fit and able. If we are older, we can end up fighting middle-aged spread, but be proactive and step in before it becomes a problem. Whatever your situation, these exercises will help to ensure you increase your levels of health and fitness.

The exercises are graded, and progress from the easiest, moving on to those of average difficulty, through to some which require more effort. How quickly you progress is entirely up to you, your degree of motivation and the time you have available.

Following this regime will not turn you into an Olympic athlete, but if you want to get fit, look fit and stay fit, then these exercises are for you.

Introduction

Why you should be fit

A person in a good state of physical fitness can deal with problems such as physical stress or fatigue better than one who is unfit. Exercise is also good for cardiac health, as well as making a positive psychological impact – if you are fit you simply feel better, and suffer fewer problems of nervous tension and anxiety.

Back pain is a major and common problem. Strengthening your back muscles is therefore a good move, as is strengthening stomach muscles to prevent sagging abdomens. You will feel better, but others will see that positive difference too. Be fit and you will enjoy life to the full.

Weight control

Weight control is about altering the relationship of body tissues – you want to decrease the amount of fat and improve your muscles. This will mean controlling your diet as well as partaking in an exercise regime. It isn't necessarily about eating less, but more about eating better.

Whatever we eat, the body deals with. Some is stored, some is used as fuel, and the rest discarded. The body stores extra calories, or fuel, as fat. A simple analogy to illustrate: If you overfill a bucket, the spare water simply spills out. The body doesn't work like that with calories. It takes in and retains whatever it is offered, however much that is in excess of what it needs, so it is logical that the more you eat the more you will store, unless you use some up by doing exercise.

So, for example, eat 4,000 calories and only use up 2,500, and the surplus 1,500 calories will be stored as fat. Every 3,500 calories consumed in excess of what is used will result in a pound of weight gained – half a bag of sugar. That soon adds up to needing a bigger size in clothing.

On the other hand, when you exercise, calories are burned off. Energy spent in this way will improve your muscle tone. Muscle, however, weighs slightly more than fat, so although your shape may improve, you will not necessarily lose weight. But muscle weight is weight which is useful.

If you do want to lose weight, then research tells us that you can do this most effectively by careful eating combined with exercise.

Physical wellbeing and fitness

Most of the human body is made up of muscles, bones and fat. You have 639 different muscles and each one:

- can produce force which can be measured
- can store energy so that it can have endurance
- can shorten itself or contract at various speeds – a process described as contraction rates
- can be stretched and then recoiled – this is because of its elasticity

These four qualities, or abilities, of your muscles are referred to as 'muscle power'. In order to function to their maximum ability the muscles need fuel on a continuous basis. It is the job of the circulatory system to carry energy in the form of oxygen from the lungs, and other necessities from the digestive system. The heart then works to force the blood carrying these things around the body to where they are needed, a process known as proving organic power.

It follows that the efficiency and capacity of your body depends upon this organic power, this is the way in which your muscles are developed, a combination of organic power and regular exercise. The level to which this muscular development can take place depends upon your body type, the food eaten and whether or not you have a medical condition which might impede it. The amount of rest and sleep you have are also involved. You can only consider yourself to be physically fit when your body is working at its most efficient level.

How fit could you be?

The genes you have inherited, combined with your health, will determine the level of fitness you can ultimately reach, that is your individual physical capacity. In most cases, however hard we train, we will never match the fitness of top Olympic athletes. We just are not made that way, but that does not mean you can't improve on your present state. The level at which you can perform right now is referred to as your 'acquired state', acquired, that is, through the physical acts you already perform as part of life.

Like a car engine, your body can perform efficiently at well below its maximum effort. Just as a car uses more fuel if driven at constant high speeds, than if driven at 30-50mph – well below what it is ultimately capable of – in the same way, your body has a better energy to work ratio if it is worked at a level below its full capacity.

It you want to avoid wasting energy you need to have a level of physical capacity which is higher than you need on a daily basis. Taking part in a regime of regular physical exercise will help you to achieve this. The capacity will increase as you gradually increase the load required from your muscles and body systems. Exercise increases both your endurance and stamina, and you build up stores of energy to use at your leisure.

Sports and other activities make a useful contribution

A balanced diet requires a little of everything and, in the same way, you need to balance physical activities so that all parts of your body are exercised. No one sport is likely to do this however, and it may be that your abdomen and back, arms and shoulders, legs or circulatory system, are not getting their fair share. But you can't take part in every sport – there is neither the time, the perceived need nor the inclination. For most people the practical answer is to take part in some sport, alongside a programme of balanced exercises. The exercises described in this book, make up just such a programme, and it only takes 12 minutes each day.

Being sensible about exercise

We have all heard about 'the burn', or exercising until it hurts. What nonsense. Pain is not necessary in order to get fit. To avoid any pain or discomfort when exercising:

- Always warm-up appropriately first before any physical activity, or other vigorous exercise.
- Begin any programme at a low level and gradually increase your activity.

Warming up correctly

Regardless of your age or level of fitness, you are at risk of straining yourself if you do not warm-up correctly. The programme outlined here includes an automatic warm-up method that depends upon both the arrangement in order of the exercises and, secondly, the way in which they are carried out.

They begin with a stretching and then loosening exercise involving large muscles. This is to be done quite slowly and gently at first, and then gradually it increases in both speed and intensity.

An example can be seen in Exercise 1. At first you are not expected to be able to touch the floor, just to push down as far as you feel able to do without causing strain. Each time this is repeated, the aim is to push just a little further. After two minutes at this, you should be able to touch the floor with relative ease and quite quickly.

Living for fitness and fitness for living

The aim of this book is to describe how you can use both exercise and diet to achieve a desired level of fitness. Just try out these exercises and make them part of your daily routine, and you will soon notice a positive difference with very little extra effort.

As well as these exercises, you could try simple things, such as getting off the bus or train a stop earlier than usual and walking at a fairly fast pace that extra bit of your journey. Whenever you can, walk instead of riding or driving, and climb those stairs instead of climbing into that lift or using the escalator.

Even drying after the bath or shower can be turned into a mini exercise if you dry yourself briskly, rather than rubbing gently.

Many of us spend hours sitting at a desk, but even then you can exercise by becoming aware of your posture. Sit up as straight as you can, without slouching or rounded shoulders. To strengthen the muscles in your shoulders and arms, place both palms flat on the desk. Bend your elbows and then push hard downwards to try and lift yourself right out of the chair for a few seconds. Doing this just three times a day takes hardly any time at all, but is just one example of using time wisely to improve your fitness.

When standing or sitting, pull in those abdomen muscles and hold them tense for about 6 seconds – count one elephant, two elephants etc., up to six, before relaxing the muscles.

Check up on yourself from time to time during the day. How is your posture? Can it be improved?

Resting, relaxing and revitalising

Your body needs exercise, but just as necessary is rest and relaxation. However, we don't all need the same amount of sleep, and you will know what you need to feel refreshed and revitalised.

If you want to sleep really well – try these tips:

- Keep the bedroom as dark as possible. You can line your curtains with blackout material relatively cheaply, and it really makes a difference if you have street lights outside, if there is a full moon, or during those early summer sunrises.

- Try not to take all your problems to bed with you, but instead think calm, positive thoughts.
- Taking mild exercise, such as walking the dog, before bed can help.
- If you are hungry, don't have a big meal, but a light snack and a warm drink will help.

If you don't relax mentally then this will affect your physical body in the form of muscular tension.

Such tension can be reduced considerably if you can teach yourself to deliberately relax muscle groups. For instance, you can relax arm muscles by holding your arms out in front of you and making tight fists and then relaxing them so that your hands are floppy. Do something similar with other muscle groups, stretching then relaxing and wriggling to relaxation.

Mentally relax by deliberately thinking of relaxing things and ignoring thoughts about anything that has troubled you in the day. Also, taking gentle exercise, such as going for a walk or playing a round of golf, will ease both physical and mental tensions.

Exercise and your heart

Your heart is a muscle and benefits from exercise. There is no evidence to suggest the heart can be harmed by a sensible exercise regime which is appropriate for your age and physical state. Instead, it is likely to improve your heart health and that of the major blood vessels. Even after a heart attack mild exercise is recommended by the medical fraternity, and for the healthy heart there are many benefits. If you are fit there will be a smaller increase in your pulse rate under physical stress, and also your heart rate will return to normal levels more quickly afterwards. A fit heart pumps more blood at rest and can increase this volume when needed. It is more efficient than an unfit heart and the small blood vessels which feed it function better. Such an efficient cardiovascular system will be able to carry oxygen and food to the muscles more effectively, as well as being able to recover better after a period of exercise.

A word of caution

Before undertaking any strenuous exercise regime, anyone with an existing medical condition should seek advice from their doctor. Depending upon the condition, particularly if it is related to the heart, intense exercise could make matters worse.

Strength, endurance and exercise

You can increase the strength and endurance of your body by undertaking exercise. Both the muscles and organs will benefit. You do need to exercise the whole body. Your arm muscles will not benefit if you concentrate only on your leg muscles, so there needs to be a balanced regime of exercise.

Your muscle strength can be measured by checking the amount of force it can exert. This depends on two things – the number of muscle fibres in use and how often the muscles receive impulses from the nervous system.

Strength goes along with endurance. The latter is about being able to keep up muscular contraction, or to repeat a particular action a number of times, such as being able to do ten leg lifts and gradually increasing this number with practice.

The fuel needed to do this, food and oxygen, is carried to the muscle by the bloodstream and this in turn depends upon the strength and efficiency of the cardiovascular system, as well as its ability to carry away waste materials as needed.

If your body is not used, it will deteriorate. For example, if you have ever broken a bone, you will have seen and felt, when the plaster cast is eventually taken off, that the muscles underneath are thinner and weaker than they were before the break happened. Unlike a machine, which will wear out with use and eventually break down, the body actually improves the more it is used. Therefore, if you exercise sensibly, more than is needed for basic everyday life, your body will increase in strength, efficiency and in its ability to endure; and your sense of wellbeing, as well as your appearance of health, will both be enhanced.

Caution

If you are in any doubt at all about your body's ability to undertake these exercise, do see your doctor first and ask their advice. Also remember that you should start slowly and gradually increase your exercises, especially if you are over 55 years of age.

Your appearance

The appearance of your body depends to a large extent upon
the frame, the skeleton beneath. This is something that obviously
cannot be changed through exercise, you can, however, alter the
amount of fat your body has and the firmness of your muscles.

We all need some fat if our bodies are to function properly. As well as
softening the bony contours, fat works to control body temperature at a constant
level and also acts as a form of storage. As well as a layer of fat beneath
the skin, each organ is lined and covered with fat, and it also interlaces the
muscles.

Except in the case of a few very particular medical conditions, most of us only
gain too much fat if we consume more calories than we need and do not work
them off.

As well as the amount of fat, muscles are also important in giving the body its
appearance. When we are young, our muscles have natural tone, but as we age
this tone can weaken and be lost. The less exercise we do, the more likely that
the muscles will become flabby and soften. If not used they weaken and shrink.

Because muscles are so important to your bodily appearance, it is important
that you are in control of them by combining a healthy diet with exercise. For
example, a thigh may be a certain measurement, but it can be made up mostly
of fat or of muscle, two very different things. The difference is up to you. A word
of warning: don't confuse good muscle tone with obviously bulky and ugly
muscles. The exercises in this book are not designed to produce a bodybuilder's
body, but simply to give you the firm muscles you need.

Diet

Often, when a person finds they have gained some weight, the
automatic reaction is to go on a diet, sometimes quite a stringent
regime. If that is what you intend to do then research one that will
best suit you and your lifestyle, allowing you the time and commitment
to follow it effectively. Remember, a diet should not be fast.

Usually, fat is added to the body at quite a slow rate. Therefore, you cannot
expect it to come off quickly. Sensible and effective weight loss takes time.
A crash diet lasts for a relatively short time, and as soon as the diet is over,
invariably, you return to your previous ways, and the fat piles on once more.
Instead, make a slight change in your diet, one you can keep up over time.
Good examples include, cutting down on the sugar in your drinks and eating
one less slice of bread, or using a smaller cereal bowl. You will hardly notice
the change after a day or two, but it will bring results over time if combined with

sufficient exercise, because over a month or so you will have eaten hundreds, or possibly thousands, of calories less than you might have done. By the time you have reached your desired weight the changes you have made will be a natural part of your daily routine, and so you are less likely to slip back into old habits.

What you can do about your fitness

Unless you are already taking part in a full-time body fitness programme for sports or athletics, then you need to participate in some form of exercise in order to be fit.

Whatever your everyday activities involve, whether you are out at work or a stay-at-home mum, none of them will give you the balanced exercise regime you need.

Some muscles get lots of exercise and others get none, or very little. Even taking part in sport may not exercise all the muscle groups evenly, and most participants in sports do not participate at a high enough level to make them properly fit. Even the sports which do provide sufficient and balanced exercise require more time and skill than most people can give to them.

Why this exercise regime was developed

Research shows quite clearly that we all need exercise, whether young or old. In the modern world there are more and more labour-saving devices available both inside and outside the home. The result is that we lead a much more sedentary life than our predecessors.

Most of us claim we want to exercise and we know it is good for us; but we do not necessarily know how to go about it, how much to do, what kind of exercise to do and how we can judge progress.

Most exercise programmes require special equipment, often only available in a gym, which makes it difficult to exercise every day.

Also, considerable time is often required, which you may not have to spare.

It is therefore obvious that what is needed is a programme which overcomes these obstacles; one which does not require special equipment or long periods of time, and which also is easy to understand, where it is clear what to do next and how to measure your progress. This is such a programme, it requires no specialist equipment, it takes less than 15 minutes a day and needs only a small amount of space.

How the regime was developed

It came about after considerable research into the physical health of women and girls. Firstly, the participants took part in several physical fitness tests. These included measuring the amount of fat carried by each person; their muscular endurance levels and strength were measured, as was the heart's response to exertion. The results of these tests were analysed and fitness levels measured.

Next, a number of different exercises were developed, and finally a series of the most effective and balanced exercises were decided upon. Various times taken by each exercise were tested until the optimum time was reached.

Several hundred women then tried out the regime, and these participants were tested regularly to see what positive effects the exercising was having. The exercises included in this book were found to be the most effective in increasing fitness.

What the plan is

There are four charts of ten exercises and these are arranged in order of difficulty. The exercises should always be carried out in the same order and for the same maximum duration. Altogether, there are 48 levels, 12 on each chart. As well as these varied exercises there are also two extra exercises on the first three charts. These are particularly for the feet and ankles because these are important in maintaining optimum good posture.

How it works

As with every other exercise regime, this one begins with easy exercises and gradually progresses in difficulty. As your fitness level improves, so the work load needed increases. This is done in two ways:

- The time taken by each level remains the same throughout, but the number of repeats necessary increases.
- At the same time as you move on from one chart to the next, the difficulty of the exercises gradually increases.

This means that you do the exercises on each chart at every level from one to twelve, but you gradually increase the number of repetitions you do. As you progress from one chart to another, the exercise described has been modified slightly to make it a little more demanding.

It is recommended that you do each exercise in turn. Do not leave any out, and do not try to go faster than is recommended.

The plan is that all the exercises on a chart can be completed within twelve minutes. It is likely, however, that at first some will take longer than others. This is perfectly normal and acceptable.

What the exercises are meant to do

These exercises will improve muscle tone and your general physical health as they:

- increase muscle tone
- increase muscular strength
- improve the amount of flexibility you have
- increase your cardiac efficiency

The first four exercises serve as a warm-up and also deal with those areas of the body most likely to be neglected, improving their flexibility and mobility. The abdominal area and the front thighs will be aided by doing exercise 5, and exercise 6 concentrates on the back of the body, the buttocks, backs of thighs and the long back muscles; whereas exercise 7 is concerned with the sides of the thighs, areas which usually do not receive sufficient exercise. Exercise 8 is designed to deal predominantly with the upper body, the arms, shoulder girdle and the chest, but will also exercise both the abdomen and the back. Exercise 9 will strengthen the muscle of the hips and your sides, but will also increase your waist's flexibility. Exercise 10 is mainly concerned with improving the condition of the heart and lungs.

There are two supplementary exercises described. One will help with posture and the other aims to add strength to your ankle joints and feet.

Chart 2

Level	Exercise											
	1	**2**	**3**	**4**	**5**	**6**	**7**	**8**	**9**	**10**	**8a**	**8b**
24	15	16	12	30	35	38	50	28	20	210	40	36
23	15	16	12	30	33	36	48	26	18	200	38	34
22	15	16	12	30	31	34	46	24	18	200	36	32
21	13	14	11	26	29	32	44	23	16	190	33	29
20	13	14	11	26	27	31	42	21	16	175	31	27
19	13	14	11	26	24	29	40	20	14	160	28	24
18	12	12	9	20	22	27	38	18	14	150	25	22
17	12	12	9	20	19	24	36	16	12	150	22	20
16	12	12	9	20	16	21	34	14	10	140	19	19
15	10	10	7	18	14	18	32	12	10	130	17	15
14	10	10	7	18	11	15	30	10	8	120	14	13
13	10	10	7	18	9	12	28	8	8	120	12	12
Minutes for each exercise	2				2	1	1	2	1	3	1	1

Recommended number of days at each level

The meaning of the charts

On the following pages you will find an explanation of what is meant on the chart pages. Check back to the chart above with each paragraph heading.

My progress

Level	Start	Finish	Notes
24			
23			
22			
21			
20			
19			
18			
17			
16			
15			
14			
13			

	Date	Height	Weight	Waist	Hips	Bust
My aim						
Start						
Finish						

Exercise

The numbers used as headings at the top of the charts are the exercises which are numbered 1 to 10. This means that the column with the heading 1 is concerned with exercise 1, etc. Each exercise is illustrated and described on the pages after each chart.

If you do wish to do the supplementary exercises, these are numbered 8A and 8B and should be fitted into your routine in-between the exercises labelled as 8 and 9.

Level

The numbers which run down the left-hand side of the charts refer to the various levels within the programme and each one refers to the line of numbers next to it under the various exercise headings. So, if you look at level 14 you will see that this tells you to carry out exercise 3 seven times, but exercise 6 should be repeated 15 times.

How far should you continue?

The physical level to which you should aim to progress depends upon your age range. The charts are aimed at the average person, so some will be capable of more than others.

Tips to help

- Don't skip a day. The more these exercises become part of your routine, the better you will be and feel.
- You may come across a level which you find very difficult to complete in anything like 12 minutes, but keep at it and progress will be seen. You are not competing with anyone else, just against your own body.
- You may find it hard to count all the steps needed in exercise 5. It is easy to lose count. Try dividing the number of steps needed by 75 or 50. Remember the answer. On a nearby surface place a row of something, such as coins or buttons, equal to the answer. Do your first set of 75 or 50 steps and move one counter. Repeat until you have moved them all.

How to make a start

It is best if the exercises can be done at the same time each day, so choose a time when you are likely to have 12 minutes to spare on a regular basis, perhaps in the early morning, although you may prefer the evening, or some other time, but whatever time you choose, try hard to stick to it *and start today*.

Maximum rates of progress

- At least one day spent on each level for those aged 20
- At least two days at each level for those aged 20-29
- At least four days at each level for those aged 30-39
- At least seven days at each level for those aged 40-49
- At least eight days at each level for those aged 50-59
- At least 10 days at each level if you are 60 or over.

If you suffer any breathlessness, or you feel sore and stiff, especially if you are in one of the older age groups, slow up your rate of progress through the levels.

Note in the box available on each chart the recommended number of days needed on a level before progressing on to the next higher level.

Your progress

The Progress Chart is there to assist you in keeping a record of the progress you are making. Make a note of the starting and finishing date of each level. Also, write down your feelings about each level. Select an achievable aim and write this on the bottom chart in the box labelled 'My Aim'. Your present measurement should be recorded on the start line. When you come to the end of each chart, make a note of your new measurements on the finish line. The changes may be quite subtle as fitness takes time and effort, so the results will not be amazing, but they will be positive. Combine these exercises with a balanced and sensible diet, and you will have success.

Fitness goals

These depend upon your age when starting the programme. Each age group has set a target they should aim to reach. The goals described are average for those taking part in each age group. Your goal then is the level of fitness which is achievable on average for someone of your age, without becoming stressed or over fatigued. As with any other average there will always be those who surpass the average and an equal number who don't quite make it. This is normal.

If you feel you really can go on further than the goals set, go for it, but on the other hand, if you find progress very difficult you need to decide to stop at a level you can maintain.

Sometimes you will reach a plateau with a particular level, but in most cases, if you persist, you will eventually succeed, usually after a few days. The goals are only meant to be guides. If, after a few days, you are not improving, you have almost certainly reached the maximum fitness as far as this exercise programme is concerned.

Caution

If, for some reason, you have a break in the programme for two weeks or more and then decide to restart, it is best to start at a level a little below the one you had reached before you stopped, perhaps even as far back as the previous chart, if you have been ill perhaps. Begin again at a level you find comfortable and then progress from there.

Instructions for following the plan

First choose the goal for your age group. Mark this in some way on the chart. Then note on the chart the minimum number of days you should spend on a level. Do not try to move on faster than the rates of progress recommended.

To begin and to progress

Level 1 starts at the base of Chart 1. Keep at this until you can do it without strain in twelve minutes or less. Once you can do this, move on to Level 2, and so on. Move on up the levels and the charts until you reach the level where you feel you have reached your full level of physical fitness or else the level which is the recommended one for your age group.

Once you reach your goal

This may seem a long way away, but you will get there. After this point has been reached you only need to exercise on three days each week in order to keep up your level of fitness.

If your age in years is	Your goal is (level)	Recommended number of days			
		Chart 1	Chart 2	Chart 3	Chart 4
7-8	30	1	1	2	-
9-10	34	1	1	2	-
11-12	38	1	1	2	3
13-14	41	1	1	2	3
15-17	44	1	1	2	3
18-19	40	1	2	3	4
20-25	35	1	2	3	-
26-30	30	2	3	5	-
31-35	26	2	4	6	-
36-40	22	4	6	-	-
41-45	19	5	7	-	-
46-50	16	7	8	-	-
51-55	11	8	-	-	-

Chart 1

Chart 1

Level	Exercise											
	1	2	3	4	5	6	7	8	9	10	8a	8b
12	9	8	10	40	26	20	30	14	14	170	18	20
11	9	8	10	40	24	18	28	13	14	160	17	18
10	9	8	10	40	22	16	26	12	12	150	16	17
9	7	7	8	36	20	14	24	10	11	140	14	15
8	7	7	8	36	18	12	20	9	10	125	13	14
7	7	7	8	36	16	12	18	8	10	115	11	12
6	5	5	7	28	14	10	16	7	8	100	10	11
5	5	5	7	28	12	8	14	6	6	90	8	9
4	5	5	7	28	10	8	10	5	6	80	7	8
3	3	4	5	24	8	6	8	4	4	70	6	6
2	3	4	5	24	6	4	6	3	3	60	5	5
1	3	4	5	24	4	4	4	3	2	50	4	3
Minutes for each exercise	2				2	1	1	2	1	3	1	1

Recommended number of days at each level ☐

My progress

Level	Start	Finish	Notes
12			
11			
10			
9			
8			
7			
6			
5			
4			
3			
2			
1			

	Date	Height	Weight	Waist	Hips	Bust
My aim						
Start						
Finish						

1 Toe-touching

Start Stand up erect with your feet 12 inches apart
and with your arms up above your head.

Bend forward so that you are touching the floor in-between
your feet. Don't worry about trying to keep your knees straight.

Return to the first position.

Count Each return to the starting position should be counted as one.

2 Knee raising

Start Stand up straight with your hands by your
sides and your feet placed together.

Raise your left knee as high as you possibly can.
Grasp your knee and shin and pull your leg in towards
your body while keeping your back as straight as
possible. Place your foot back on the floor.

Repeat this with your other leg and
continue with the legs alternately.

Count A raise of first the left and then the right knee counts as one.

CHART 1

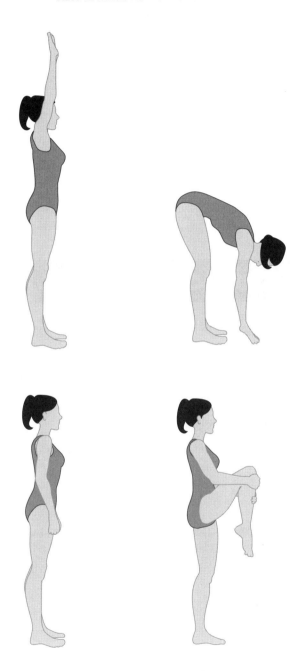

3 Lateral bending

Start Stand up straight with your hands by your sides. Your feet should be about 12 inches apart. While keeping your back straight, bend to the left sideways and slide your hand on that side as far down your leg as possible.

Repeat to the right side.

Count A bend first to the left and then to the right counts as one.

CHART 1

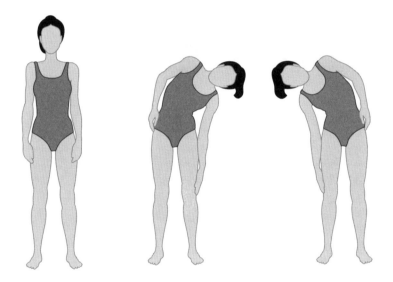

4 Arm circling

Start Stand up straight with your arms at your sides and your feet a foot apart.

Make circles as big as you can with your left arm and then your right one.

Half your total of circles with each arm should be forward and half backwards.

Count A full circle counts as one.

CHART 1

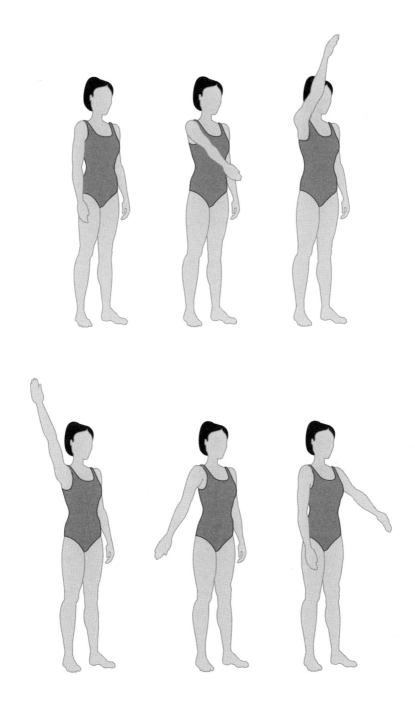

5 Partial sit-ups

Start   Lie down on your back with your arms at your sides
and keep your legs straight. Raise your head and
shoulder girdle up off the floor until your heels
are visible. Lower your head back down.

Count   Each of these partial sit-ups counts as one.

6 Raising the chest and leg raising

Start   Lie face down with your arms along your sides and your hands
beneath your thighs and with the palms of your hands pressed
along your thighs. Keeping your legs straight, raise your
left leg as far as you can and with your head and shoulders
raised at the same time. Lower yourself to the floor. Repeat
this using the other leg and continue alternating the legs.

Count   Each raise of a leg counts as one.

CHART 1

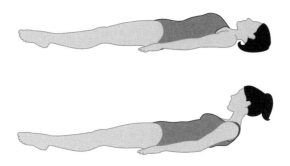

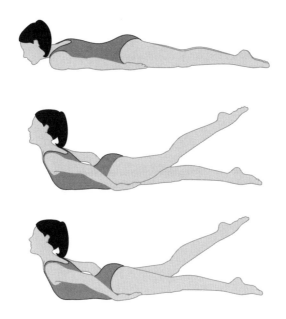

7 Side leg raising

Start Lie on your side with your legs straight. Your upper arm is used for balance and the lower arm is stretched along the floor above your head. Raise the upper leg about 18-24 inches in the air. Lower it to the start position.

Count Each raise of a leg counts as one. Do half the required count with one leg and then roll over and use your other leg for the remaining count.

CHART 1

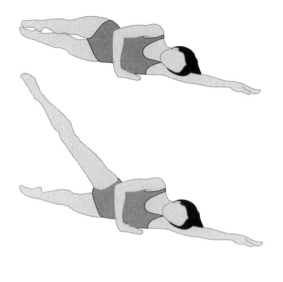

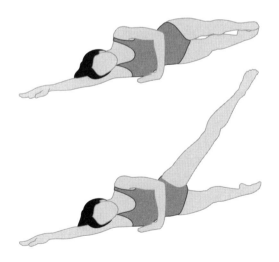

8 Push-ups

Start Lie with your face down towards the floor. Your legs should be straight and your hands should be placed underneath your shoulders as in the diagram. Keeping your knees and hands in contact with the floor, push your body upwards. Sit back onto your heels. Lower your body back down to the floor.

Count Each time you lower yourself back down, count one.

CHART 1

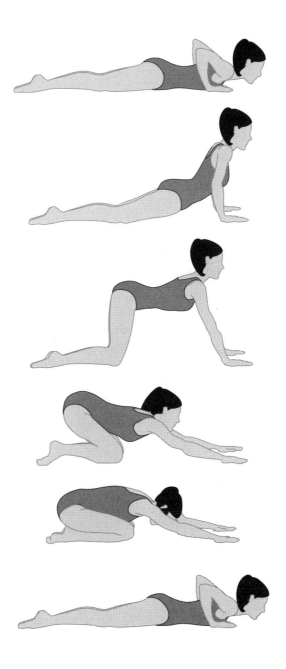

9 Leg lifting

Start Lie on your back with your arms by your sides and your hands palm side down. Raise your right leg until it is at right angles with the floor, or as near to this as you can possibly do. Lower the leg and repeat with your left leg. Continue, alternating your limbs.

Count Raising first one leg and then the other counts as one.

CHART 1

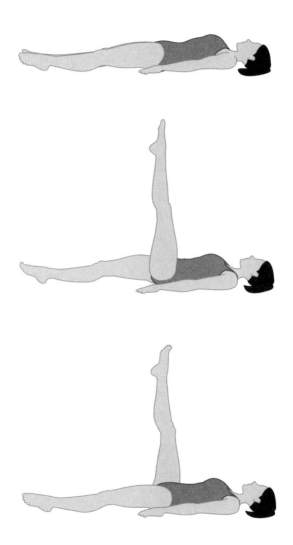

10 Running and hopping

This combines two separate actions

Start Stand up straight with your arms by your sides and your feet placed closely together. Beginning with your left leg, run on the spot. Your feet should be raised at least four inches above the floor with each movement. Don't just move your heels backwards, but also move your knees forwards.

Count Each time you lift your left foot count one. Only these running steps add to your count.

After counting each fifty do ten hops, which means lifting both feet right off the floor together. You should try to raise yourself at least four inches off the floor.

CHART 1

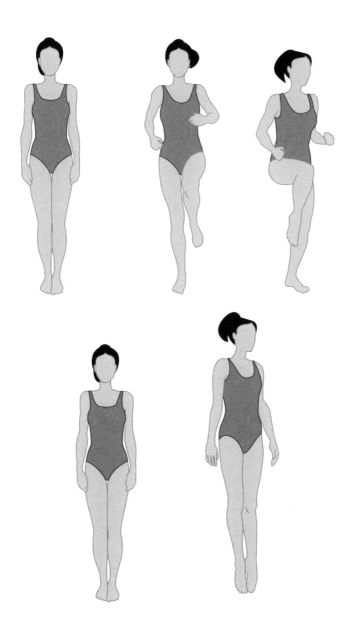

Chart 2

Chart 2

Level	Exercise											
	1	2	3	4	5	6	7	8	9	10	8a	8b
24	15	16	12	30	35	38	50	28	20	210	40	36
23	15	16	12	30	33	36	48	26	18	200	38	34
22	15	16	12	30	31	34	46	24	18	200	36	32
21	13	14	11	26	29	32	44	23	16	190	33	29
20	13	14	11	26	27	31	42	21	16	175	31	27
19	13	14	11	26	24	29	40	20	14	160	28	24
18	12	12	9	20	22	27	38	18	14	150	25	22
17	12	12	9	20	19	24	36	16	12	150	22	20
16	12	12	9	20	16	21	34	14	10	140	19	19
15	10	10	7	18	14	18	32	12	10	130	17	15
14	10	10	7	18	11	15	30	10	8	120	14	13
13	10	10	7	18	9	12	28	8	8	120	12	12
Minutes for each exercise	2				2	1	1	2	1	3	1	1

Recommended number of days at each level ☐

My progress

Level	Start	Finish	Notes
24			
23			
22			
21			
20			
19			
18			
17			
16			
15			
14			
13			

	Date	Height	Weight	Waist	Hips	Bust
My aim						
Start						
Finish						

1 Toe-touching

Start Stand straight with your arms above your head and with your feet a foot apart. Bend forward so that you can touch the floor between your feet. Bob up and then down, repeating the floor-touching once more.

Count Each time you return to the 'arms above the head position' counts as one.

2 Knee raising

Start Stand up straight with your feet kept together and with your arms straight at your sides. Raise your left knee as high up as possible. Grasp the knee and the shin with both hands. Pull the leg in towards the body, but keep your back straight. Place your foot back on the floor. Repeat with the other leg and continue alternating the legs used.

Count Raising first one knee and then the other counts as one.

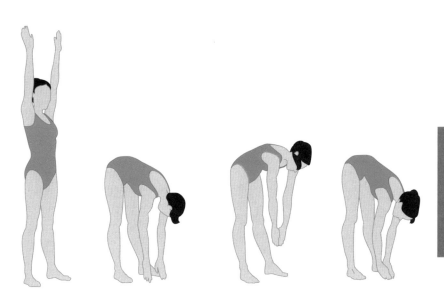

CHART 2

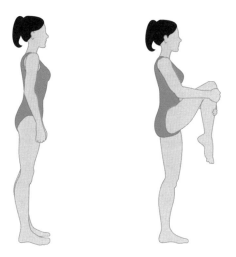

3 *Lateral bending*

Start Stand straight with your arms by your sides and your feet placed a foot apart. Keeping your back as straight as possible, bend from waist level to the left side, while sliding your left hand as far down the outer side of the leg as possible. Bob up a few inches and then bend once more. Return to your starting stance and repeat on the alternate side. Continue with a bend to each side in turn.

Count A bend first to the left and then to the right counts as one.

4 *Arm circling*

Start Stand straight with your arms at your sides and your feet placed a foot apart. Using both arms at the same time, make as large backwards circles as you possibly can. After you have done half the number of repetitions required, then change over to forward circles.

Count Each complete circle counts as one.

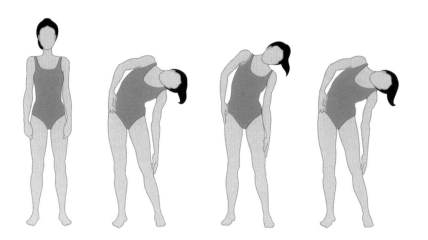

CHART 2

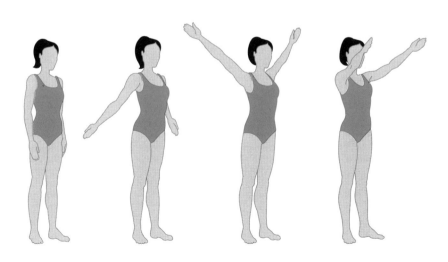

5 *Rocking sit-ups*

Start Lie down on your back with your arms over your head. Your knees should be bent so that the soles of your feet are flat on the floor. Swing your arms forward while, at the same time, thrusting your feet forward, moving into a sitting position. Now stretch forward and touch the tips of your toes with your fingers. Go back to the start position.

Count Every time you return to your starting position, you count one.

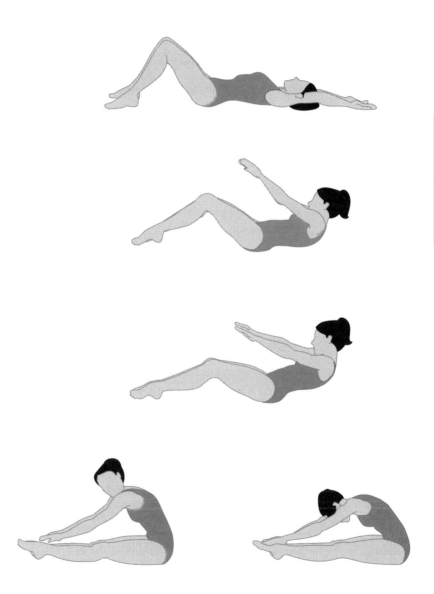

CHART 2

6 Leg and chest raising

Start Lie on your front with your arms at your sides, and your hands should have their palms pressing on the thighs. Keep your legs straight while raising your legs, together with your head and shoulders, as far upwards as possible. Relax and go back to your original position.

Count Each time you return to your starting pose, count one.

7 Side leg raising

Start Lie on your side. You should keep your legs straight and you should have your lower arm stretched above your head. You use the other arm to improve your balance. Raise your upper leg until it is at right angles with the floor, or as near to this as you can manage. Bring your leg back down.

Count Each time you lift your leg up, count one. For half of the required count use your left leg, and then roll over and use the other leg for the rest of the count.

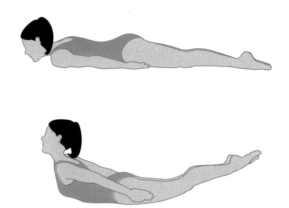

CHART 2

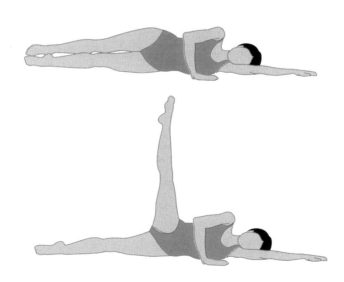

8 Knee push-ups

Start Begin by lying face down on the floor with your hands placed under your shoulders and your legs kept straight and close together. Push down with your hands until your arms are straight and your torso is off the floor. Your knees should remain in touch with the floor throughout. You should aim to keep your body in as straight a line as possible. Let yourself return to the starting position.

Count Each return to the flat position counts as one.

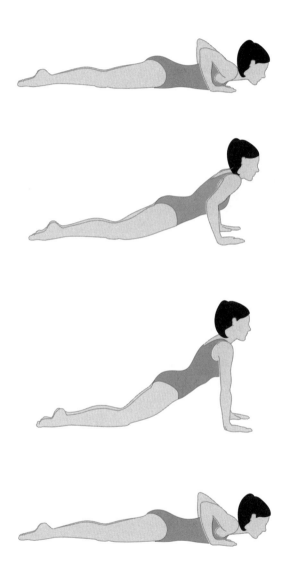

CHART 2

9 Leg overs

Start   Lie on your back with your arms stretched out sideways and your legs straight and together. Raise your right leg to the upright position and then drop it down across your body, as if trying to touch your fingers with the tips of your toes. Raise your leg up again and then return it to the starting position. Repeat this action with your other leg. Your shoulders should stay in contact with the floor and your body should be as straight as possible all the time, and so should your leg.

Count   Each time you return to the first position counts as one.

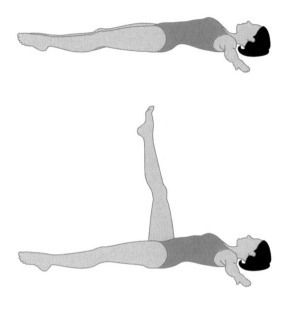

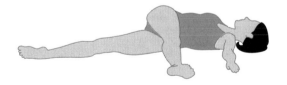

CHART 2

10 *Running and stride jumping*

Start Stand straight up with your feet placed together and with your hands placed by your sides. Beginning with your left leg, followed by the right, raise each foot at least four inches from the ground.

Count Each time your left foot is raised up, this counts as one.

After a count of 50, carry out 10 stride jumps. These begin with your hands at your sides and with your feet together. Jump so that the feet, when you land, are about 18 inches apart. When you jump, raise up your arms to the sides to the height of your shoulders. Then jump again so that your feet come together again and your arms are back at your sides. These two jumps together count as one.

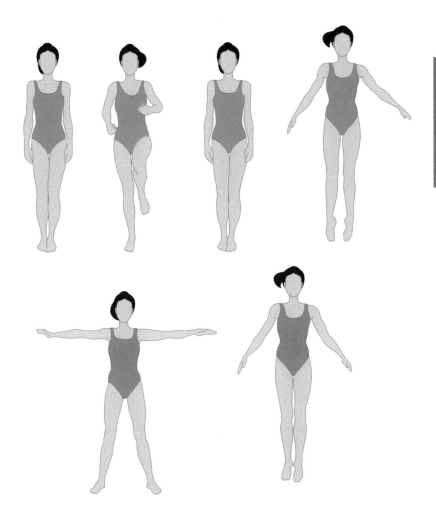

CHART 2

Chart 3

Chart 3

Level	Exercise											
	1	2	3	4	5	6	7	8	9	10	8a	8b
36	15	22	18	40	42	40	60	40	20	240	32	38
35	15	22	18	40	41	39	60	39	20	230	30	36
34	15	22	18	40	40	38	58	37	19	220	29	34
33	13	20	16	36	39	36	58	35	19	210	27	33
32	13	20	16	36	37	36	56	34	18	200	25	31
31	13	20	16	36	35	34	56	32	16	200	24	30
30	12	18	14	30	33	33	54	30	15	190	23	28
29	12	18	14	30	32	31	54	29	14	180	21	26
28	12	18	14	30	31	30	52	27	12	170	20	25
27	10	16	12	24	29	30	52	25	11	160	19	23
26	10	16	12	24	27	29	50	23	9	150	17	21
25	10	16	12	24	26	28	48	22	8	140	16	20
Minutes for each exercise	2				2	1	1	2	1	3	1	1

Recommended number of days at each level

My progress

Level	Start	Finish	Notes
36			
35			
34			
33			
32			
31			
30			
29			
28			
27			
26			
25			

	Date	Height	Weight	Waist	Hips	Bust
My aim						
Start						
Finish						

1 Toe-touching

Start   Stand straight with your feet placed so that they are about 16 inches apart. Bend over and touch the floor to the left of your left foot with both hands; bob up and then back down to touch the floor between your feet; bob again and then touch the floor on the outside of your right foot. Stand up straight again in your starting position.

Count   Each time you stand up straight again counts as one.

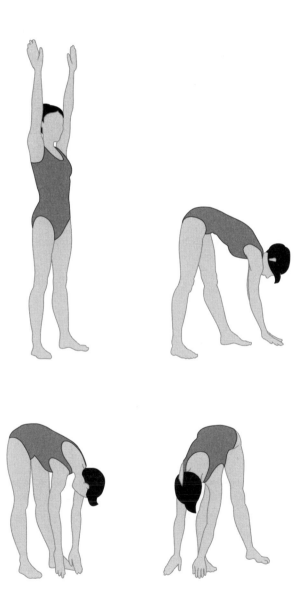

CHART 3

2 Knee raising

Start Stand straight with your feet placed together and with your hands by your sides. Raise your left knee as high as possible and then grasp it, and your shin, with your hands and then draw it close to your body. With your back kept straight, lower your foot to the floor. Now repeat this action with your other knee. Continue to the required count, alternating the legs.

Count Raising first the left and then the right leg counts as one.

3 Lateral bending

Start Stand straight up with your right arm lifted up and over the head, but keep your elbow bent. Your feet should be a foot apart. Keeping your spine straight, bend from the waist to the left side. Press towards the left with your right arm, while at the same time sliding your left hand as far down on your leg as possible. Return to your first position and then change over your arm positions before continuing to the right side. Return to the beginning.

Count A bend first to the left and then to the right counts as one.

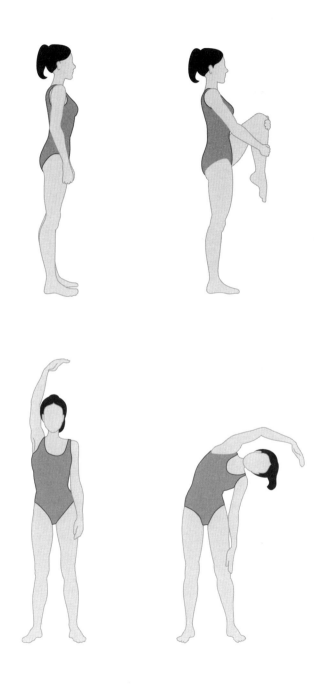

CHART 3

4 Arm circling

Start Begin by standing up straight with your arms by your sides and your feet placed about a foot apart. Use both arms to make large circles with one arm following the other in a windmill pattern. Half the required number of repetitions should be carried out moving forward and half by swinging the arms backwards.

Count A full circle of both arms makes a count of one.

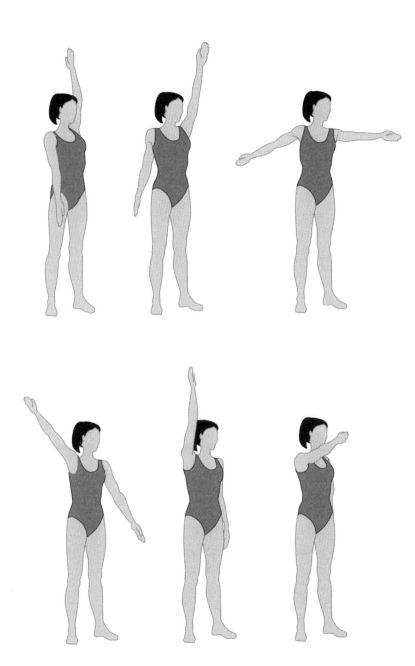

CHART 3

5 Sit-ups

Start Lie flat on your back with your legs placed together and straight, and with your arms close by your sides. While keeping your back as straight as you possibly can, raise yourself to the sitting position. Slide both hands along your legs towards your toes and touch them. Return to the original position.

Count Each time you lie back down counts as one.

6 Chest and leg raising

Start Lie down on your front with your arms stretched out to the sides at shoulder level. Your legs should be placed together and straight. Lift up your whole upper body, together with your legs, which should be as straight as possible. Return to the initial position.

Count Each return to the first position counts as one.

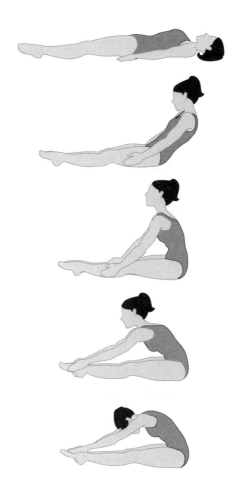

CHART 3

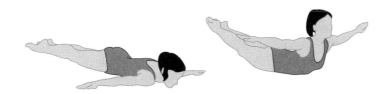

7 Side leg raising

Start   Lie on your side with your legs straight. Your upper arm
should be used to give you balance while your lower
arm is placed above your head on the floor. Lift up your
upper leg until it is at right angles with the floor. Lower
the leg to its original position. Do half the number of
counts with one leg and the rest with the other.

Count   Each time you raise your leg, count one.

8 Elbow push-ups

Start   Lie down facing the floor. Keep your legs together and straight.
Your elbows should be straight under your shoulders, so that
they are at right angles to the floor. Keep your head raised
throughout. Your forearms should be placed along the floor
and your hands should be clasped together. Lift your body up
from the floor, keeping it as straight as you can. When you
are in the raised position, your body will maintain a straight
line and your toes, elbows and forearms keep in contact with
the floor surface. Now lower yourself to the original position.

Count   Count one each time you return to the lower position.

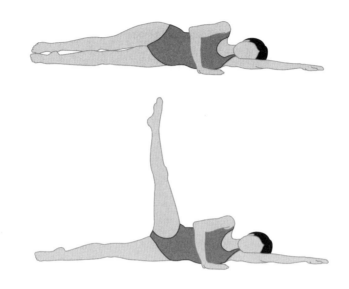

CHART 3

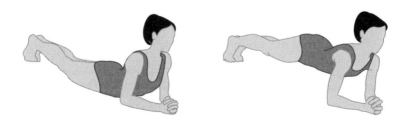

9 Legs over with tuck

Start Lie on your back with your arms stretched out sideways and with the palms pointing downwards. Your legs should be straightened and kept together. Lift up both your legs towards your body into a tuck position. With your shoulders kept in contact with the floor, lower your legs first to the left, and then to the right. The legs should remain in the tuck position. Return your knees to the starting perpendicular position.

Count Each time you return to the beginning counts as one.

10 Run and half knee bends

Start Stand up straight with your arms by your sides and your legs placed together. Beginning with your left foot, raise each foot in turn, lifting them at least 6 inches up from the floor.

Count Each time your left foot touches the floor counts as one. After each fifty counts do ten half knee bends.

Half knee bends
Half knee bends start with hands on hips, feet together, body erect. Bend at knees and hips, lowering body until thigh and calf form an angle of about 110 degrees. Do not bend knees past a right angle. Keep back straight. Return to starting position.

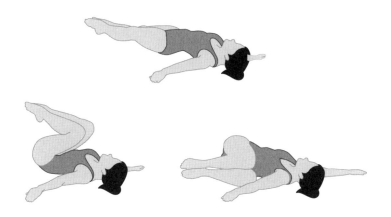

CHART 3

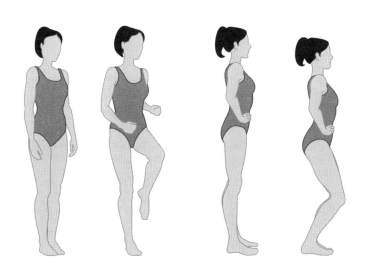

Chart 4

Chart 4

Level	Exercise									
	1	**2**	**3**	**4**	**5**	**6**	**7**	**8**	**9**	**10**
48	15	26	15	32	48	46	58	30	16	230
47	15	26	15	32	45	45	56	27	15	220
46	15	26	15	32	44	44	54	24	14	210
45	13	24	14	30	42	43	52	21	13	200
44	13	24	14	30	40	42	50	19	13	190
43	13	24	14	30	38	40	48	16	12	175
42	12	22	12	28	35	39	46	13	10	160
41	12	22	12	28	32	38	44	11	9	150
40	12	22	12	28	30	38	40	9	8	140
39	10	20	10	26	29	36	38	8	7	130
38	10	20	10	26	27	35	36	7	6	115
37	10	20	10	26	25	34	34	6	5	100
Minutes for each exercise	2				2	1	1	2	1	3

Recommended number of days at each level

My progress

Level	Start	Finish	Notes
48			
47			
46			
45			
44			
43			
42			
41			
40			
39			
38			
37			

	Date	Height	Weight	Waist	Hips	Bust
My aim						
Start						
Finish						

1 Toe-touching

Start Stand upright with your hands over your head and with your feet about 16 inches apart. Bend down to touch the floor to the left of your left foot. Bob up and then touch the floor between your two feet. Bob up again and then touch the floor between the feet once more. Bob up and then bend so that you can touch the floor on the right of your right foot. Return to the upright position.

Count Count one each time you return to the upright position.

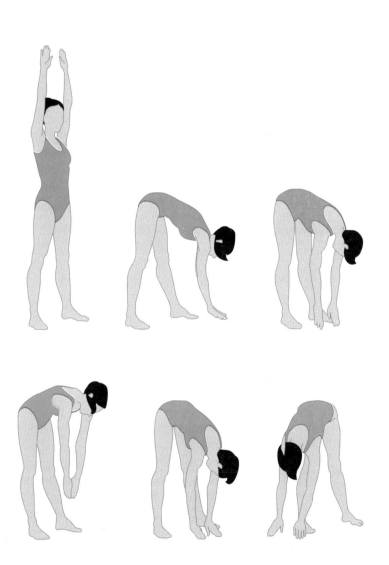

CHART 4

2 Knee raising

Start Stand upright with your feet together and with your hands by your sides. Lift your left knee as high as you can, holding your knee and shin with your hands. Keep your back straight, while pulling the knee in towards the body. Place the foot back on the floor. Do this with the other leg. Continue to alternate the legs until you reach the required number.

Count One raising of both knees, one after the other, counts as one.

3 Lateral bending

Start Stand straight up with your feet a foot apart. Extend your hand over your head with the arm bent at the elbow. Keep your back straight while bending sideways from the waist towards the left. Slide your left hand gradually as far as you can while also pressing to the left with your right hand. Bob a few inches towards the upright and then press to the left once more. Return to the original position and swap over the position of your arms. Repeat on the right side. Alternate from right to left as many times as needed.

Count One set of bends to the left and right counts as one.

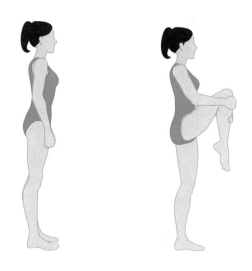

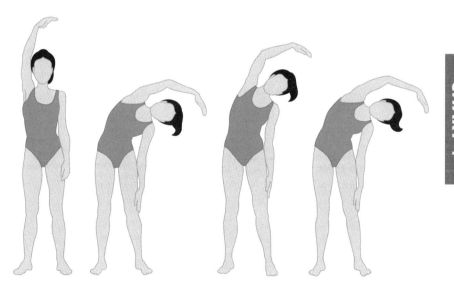

CHART 4

4 Arm flinging

Start   Stand up straight with your feet a foot apart. Your upper
arms should be at shoulder height, extended, but with
the elbows bent and your fingertips touching in front of
you. Do not let your elbows drop while you press them
backwards and upwards. Bring your arms back to the
first position and then fling your arms out and back and
up as far as you can. Go back to the first position.

Count   After each arm fling, count one.

5 Sit-ups

Start   Lie on your back with your legs together and lying straight,
and place your hands under your head. Move into a
sitting position while keeping your feet on the floor and
your back straight. Lower the body back onto the floor.

Count   Each time you lie back down, count one.

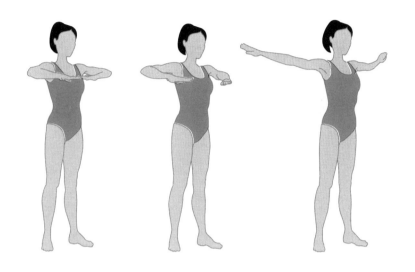

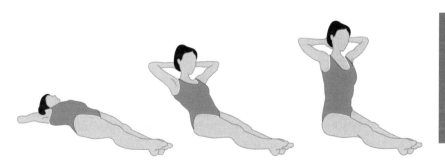

CHART 4

6 Raising the chest and legs

Start Lie down facing the floor with your hands behind your head and your legs together and straight. Lift up your legs and upper body as far off the floor as you can while you keep your legs in a straight position. Return to the initial position.

Count Each time you return to the first position, count one.

7 Side leg raising

Start With your right side in contact with the floor and with your arm straight, support your body weight on the side of your foot and your hand. You may need to use your other hand to give you extra balance. Raise your left leg to a position where it is parallel to the floor surface. Lower the leg once more. Repeat for half the count and then swap sides and do the other half.

Count Each leg raise and return counts as one.

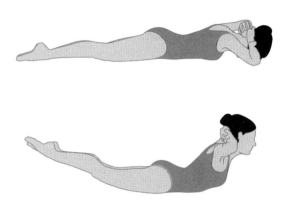

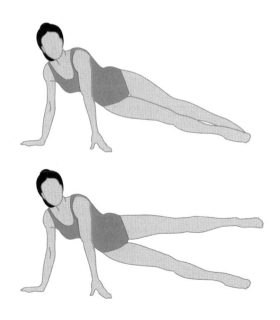

CHART 4

8 Push-ups

Start Lie on your front. Keep your legs together and straight, but with your toes turned under and with your hands directly underneath your shoulders. Push upwards with the toes and hands until your arms are straight and fully extended. Still keeping your legs and body in one straight line, lower yourself until your chest touches the ground once more.

Count Each time you return your chest to the floor counts as one.

9 Straight leg overs

Start Begin by lying down on your back with your arms stretched out to the sides and your palms pointing down to the floor. Your legs should be together and kept straight. Lift both legs until they are at right angles with the floor, at the same time keeping them straight and close together. Lower your legs to the left side, trying to reach your left hand with your toes and twisting from the waist. Lift your legs to the perpendicular position once more and then over to the right. Lift them back up to the upright and then lower them to the starting position.

Count Each time you place your legs back on the floor, count one.

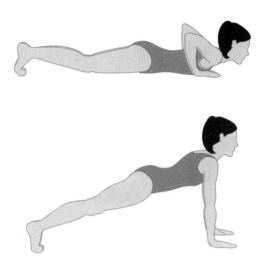

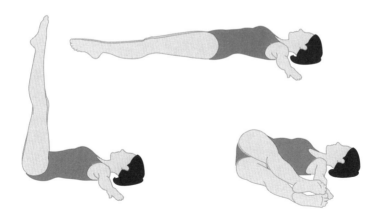

CHART 4

10 Run with semi-squat jumps

Start   Stand up straight with your arms by your sides and with your feet placed closely together. Beginning with your left foot, run on the spot, lifting your leg at least 6 inches above the floor.

Count   Every time your left foot returns to the floor counts as one.

After you have counted to 50 carry out 10 semi-squat jumps. These are done by dropping into a half crouch with your arms kept straight and with your hands placed on your knees. One foot should be placed just in front of the other and your back should remain as straight as is possible. Jump up into an upright position so that your feet leave the floor and your back is straight. Before you land once more, reverse the position of your two feet. Go back into the crouch position and repeat for a count of ten.

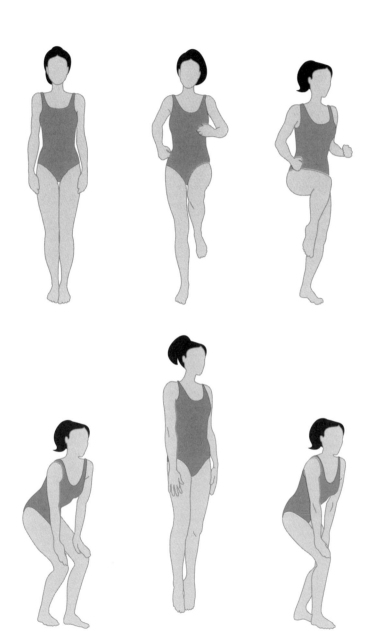

Extra exercises

On the remaining pages there are exercises which help your posture and also your ankles and feet. If you decide to include these in your programme then fit them in-between exercises 8 and 9. They should be numbered as 8A and 8B.

8a Feet and ankles exercise

Start Sit on the floor with your legs out in front of you. Your feet should be about 6 inches apart. Your feet should be relaxed and you should place your hands behind you to give you support. Press your toes down so that they are as far away from your body as they can be. Now reverse this, bringing your toes up towards your body, hooking your feet as much as possible. Relax.

Count Each time you push, hook and then relax counts as one.

8b Body posture

Start Sit down on the floor. Your knees should be bent and the soles of your feet flat on the floor. Clasp your knees with your hands, bend your head forward and sit in a relaxed state. Now straighten up and, at the same time, pull in your abdominal muscles tight for a few seconds. Relax.

Count Each time you relax counts as one.

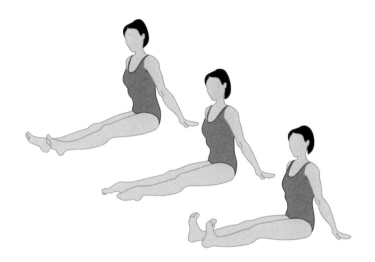

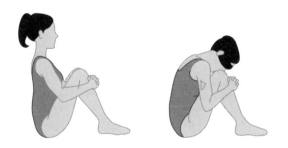

8a *Feet and ankles*
exercise

Start   Sit down on the floor with your legs straight out in front of you and your heels in contact with the floor, about 14 inches apart. Your hands should be giving you support by being placed behind your body. Move your feet so that your toes describe large circles. Press them out and around and then in towards the body. For half the count move your feet in one direction and for the second half of the count, reverse this direction.

Count   Each full circle made by your toes counts as one.

8b *Posture*

Start   Lie on your back, relaxed, and with your knees bent up and with the soles of your feet on the floor. Your arms should be placed at the sides just a few inches from your body. Tighten the muscles of your back and abdomen, pushing your lower back down towards the ground. Relax.

Count   Each time you relax in the starting position, count one.

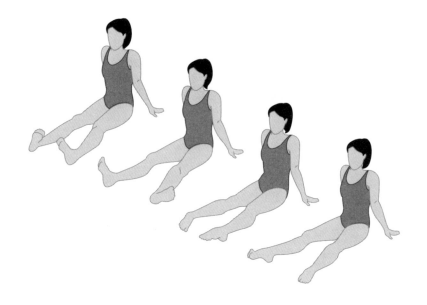

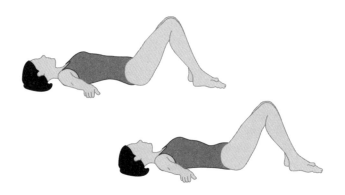

8a Ankles and feet

Start Stand straight, with your feet about a foot apart and with your arms by your sides. Push down on your toes, raising your heels up off the floor. Lower your heels back down. Next, roll your feet so that the outside of each foot is in contact with the floor. Now move them so that the outside edge of each foot is up off the floor. Return your feet to the straight position.

Count Each time you straighten up your feet, count one.

8b Posture

Start Lie down on your back. Your legs should be relaxed and placed straight together. Your arms should be relaxed and at your sides. Relax the muscles in your upper body. Tighten up the muscles in your back and abdomen, and press your lower back towards the floor. Relax again into the starting position.

Count Returning to the starting position counts as one.

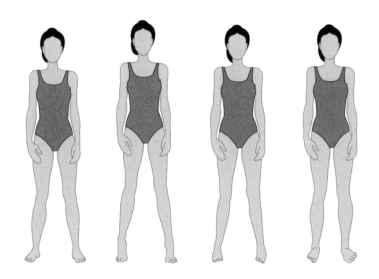

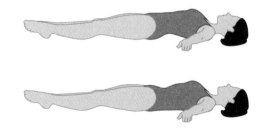